Copyright 2017 Enlighten Medical Media, LLC

All Rights Reserved. No part of this publication may be reproduced, distributed, or transmitted in any form or by any means, including photocopying, recording, or other electronic or mechanical methods, without the prior written permission of the publisher, except in the case of brief quotations embodied in critical reviews and certain other noncommercial uses permitted by copyright law. For permission requests, write to the publisher via email: requests@pastartup.co

WRITING YOUR PA SCHOOL APPLICATION ESSAY

PASTARTUP.CO

To My Girls:
Jana, Paisley, Majil, and Juniper

I Love You!

FOREWORD

I interact with pre-PA and pre-health students regularly, and one of the most common things I'm asked is about how to write a good essay. Over the years, competition has gotten more and more intense, so it's more important now than ever to write a good essay. What's amazing is the impact your essay can have on your PA school application; it's looked at as one piece of the application when it should be viewed as the main piece of the application.

I'm one of you—I was a pre-PA student once, so I know what it's like to want to write something great to stand out. Staring at a blank screen is intimidating, so this short workbook is designed to get the ideas flowing. The first half is to get some things out of your head and on paper, then bring it all together with some rules and a "recipe" for an ideal flow of your narrative at the last half.

A single blog post or video doesn't get deep enough to be helpful since crafting a good essay takes patience, some effort, a little personal insight, and commitment to make it a priority in the application process.

I'd love to hear your feedback: comments, criticisms, or even a quick "hello", so please shoot me an email or tweet at your convenience and let me know what you think of this workbook—good, bad, or ugly!

And definitely let me know when you get accepted into school, we'll do a virtual toast to your success.

I'm excited for us to be colleagues in the near future.

Chris Darst, MPAS, PA-C
PA Startup
chris@pastartup.co
Twitter: @PAStartupDOTco
Facebook: @PAStartup.co

TABLE OF CONTENTS

Introduction 5
The Good News 9
First Things First 11
My Experience 13
Final Words Before
We Construct Greatness 15
Getting Started 17
Motivation 21
Formative Experiences 25
Your Turn 31
Competition 35
10 Key Points To Remember 37
Assembly of Your Statement 41
Editing 47

Bonus Interview Questions 49
About the Author 50
Disclaimer 51
Notes 52

INTRODUCTION

All PA school applicants have several things in common: you all have taken the same prerequisites. You all have submitted grades to CASPA. You all have competitive test scores. Your personal and professional references are all exceedingly glowing. Am I right?

When comparing these similar components of applications, admissions committees all across the country basically have a stack of very similar applicants. There might be subtle differences in grades, GPA, volunteer hours…but not that much…

So how do you stand out to the admissions committee?

Your essay.

CASPA calls it an essay, but it's much more than that. It can go by many other terms: personal statement, personal narrative, persuasion essay. Your essay is possibly the most important independent variable of your application to PA school. Don't think of this as something that's scary or intimidating, but rather—think of it as an opportunity.

Even though CASPA calls it an essay, let's refer to it as a "personal statement". It's personal because you should obviously be writing about you, not some global health concept or general statement about the PA profession. Specifically, it's why you're interested in being a PA.

It's a "statement" because it's not a question, you're stating that which is true about yourself. You're telling your audience facts about why you want to/need to become a PA. When it's presented this way, you can see its potential.

If calling it an "essay" might undermine its importance, then CASPA makes it even worse by giving this vague direction: "Please explain why you are interested in being a Physician Assistant."

There you go…at 5000 characters max, it sure doesn't look like your window of opportunity.

Based on CASPA's direction, you might be tempted to write a few sentences….but if you stop there, you're missing your chance to stand out from the other applicants.

To make matters worse, it's surprisingly hard to write about yourself. You're used to writing research papers and citing sources, but when you're forced to write about yourself, its uncomfortable and takes much more effort than you realize.

I've seen students with high GPAs and poor personal statements get passed up for a seat in a class. I've seen students with a lower GPA but compelling personal statements snagging one of those coveted seats.

Which one do you want to be? It's a difference maker. So make sure it's exceptional.

Your grades are what they are; it's impossible to go back and change them.

If you chose your references wisely (and I'm sure you did), they will represent you well. Unfortunately, so will everyone else's.

Your next victory after application submission is an interview if all goes well, but between now and then, you first have to be selected from the applicant pool. Your personal statement is the one major differentiator at this point that can separate you from other applicants you're competing against. It's your opportunity to add personality to the prerequisites and transcripts; when done well it can catapult you to the top of the applicant pool.

I want this workbook to be as helpful as possible for you. By the end of this book, I want you to be able to write the best personal narrative you possibly can. However, I want to be upfront with you: this isn't a guarantee that you will get an interview. Much of the application process is subjective to the person reading the applications. But there are components that, when put together in the proper order, can make your personal statement shine. You have it in you, you just need to get it out in an orderly fashion and prove to the committee why they NEED you in the class.

Your personal statement can't make up for poor grades or make up for missing prerequisites. What it can do, however, is provide an irresistible representation of who you are to the application committee.

THE GOOD NEWS

You know what? You're unique. Why do you want to dilute that uniqueness by conforming to a "safe" illustration in your personal statement?

Too often, applicants play it safe. Our instinct is to write in vague sweeping terms in an attempt to appeal to a wider audience. We want to seem well balanced and not too shocking, so we tone it down so as not to alienate our readers. Unfortunately, what ends up happening is you're left with a very boring personal statement.

I've read some statements that talk about "learning as a young child the value of altruism" (barf) and how someone has "a strong, unwavering desire to help the poor and needy" (dry heave). While these statements might be true, DON'T BLEND IN! There are some common inherent draws to the medical profession: helping people, making a difference, being a resource...but we ALL have those in common, so what unique reasons make YOU want to be a PA?

Think of it this way: if you're on the applications committee, do you want to read 300 personal statements that all paint a rosy picture of selfless caring applicants who promise to put patients first? I think that's a noble goal for all of us, but I don't want to read it a million times.

When I was on the admissions committee for a local PA school, I was shocked at the number of personal statements that were written to everyone who could possibly be on the admissions committee—young and hip (like me of course!) to an aging semi-retired physician to a college professor. They all seemed to take the same angle: gaining invaluable experience during 4 hours at a homeless shelter or something similar, and how they were totally not selfish, and how they weren't after financial success but rather wanted to be a servant in the medical field. After the 4th or 5th of the day, I honestly stopped reading. "Ok, I get it...based on what I've read, all these people sound like the most selfless people ever... but what makes them unique? All I've learned is that everyone will be helping little old ladies cross the street at every opportunity. Good for you." (Too harsh? I wouldn't like, let the old ladies get hit by a car, but I'm also not constantly looking to save the day, you know!?)

Not to sound cheesy, but there is no one in the world like you. No one has had your upbringing, your experiences, or your personal motivation. No one has walked in your shoes; no one has seen the things you've seen through your eyes. You bring a one-of-a-kind viewpoint.

Do you see what I'm getting at?

Simply: don't make it lame.

Don't be boring.

There is a "system" to a good personal statement. There is a "recipe" of sorts to writing a good statement, but the content is more important than following a recipe. We need to tease out the content first, then structure it to fit together, illustrating the awesomeness that is you, and bam: a winning personal statement.

FIRST THINGS FIRST

Remember your audience. Keep in mind: admissions committees are looking for students who can succeed and thrive in their programs. They need students who can not only handle the intellectual side of PA school, but be able to have good rapport with preceptors/medical community and solid bedside manner with patients. This is why the ideal applicant is described as "well rounded". "Well rounded" doesn't mean boring though...! You just have to illustrate that you're unique, you deserve a seat, and you can handle the rigors of PA training.

PA school is intense, so you obviously need to be able to handle the information that is flying at you with a dizzying pace. But once you have that information, can you apply it?

Can you communicate the information to providers, patients, and families? We all know someone who is very smart, but can't hold a conversation with others...they lack the skill of interpersonal communication. You have to have more than smarts as a PA, you also need to have strong interpersonal skills. The first chance you get to showcase this is your personal statement.

Students with superior interpersonal communication skills build good relationships with preceptors and others in the community, which represents the program well, which increases the community perception of the program and thus drives more applicants.

PA schools obviously want to train strong members of the medical community, but they also want to attract the best and the brightest to keep a flow of incoming students. (Don't get me started on PA school tuition...!!)

Remember this as you work your way through the application process: it's not solely about grades but also being a well-rounded individual.

MY EXPERIENCE

I wrote my first personal narrative much the same as I wrote a number of papers in high school. I used big words, referenced "hot button" topics in medicine at the time, and wrote what I thought the committee wanted to read.

Did you catch that? I wrote what I thought they wanted to read rather than what represented me.

I talked about the honor and personal satisfaction I'd get as a PA and how I could provide cost-effective medical care. I pretty much thought I nailed it.

Then I sent it to my dad, a physician, to read and review.

I was expecting a "killed it son, that's my boy" But instead I got this in an email response:

"Pretty good. I could do an "English teacher"-type rewrite if you want. –Dad"

That was it.

No "BINGO you stud, you made me cry with laughter and weep with emotion!" or "holy guacamole, your wife is lucky to be married to such a confident but humble and selfless saint!"

He didn't even say it was good, no, he said it was "pretty good". That's like the judge of a cooking show take a bite of what you've made and shrug: "Meh. Not bad." As in, "doesn't stink".

Your goal is NOT to merely avoid stinking. Your goal for your statement to be AWESOME.

My feelings were hurt, but I couldn't argue with him. It was pretty beige. Not exciting, not moving…just…there.

So, much like the night before a paper was due in college, I hit Cmd-A (I'm a Mac user!) and deleted it. I started over from scratch. I closed my eyes and wrote what I wanted the admissions committee to know, not what I thought they wanted to hear. I illustrated why the committee needed to choose me for a seat in their class.

I hit some high points (meeting my wife) and some low points (being in and out of college). I didn't use big words but rather was conversational (without contractions or f-bombs, of course) as though I was speaking directly to the committee.

When I sent it to my dad again, I got the response I was originally after:

"Whoa. Knocked my socks off; nice work."

Boom shakka lakka.

Don't Cmd-A -delete anything you've done so far…hang onto it. We can possibly draw from it later.

But for now, grab a pen and get ready to take some notes, pick your brain, and take the pressure off this process. This isn't all going to go into the final product, but I want you to get some great stuff down and we can pick from the best at the end.

FINAL WORDS BEFORE WE CONSTRUCT EXCELLENCE

Don't forget: PA school seats are competitive. There are a lot of applications for a limited number of seats. This isn't like picking a kickball team on a playground where it's just fun to get to play. This is a fight. You're fighting for your seat in the class. You need to throw the best punches you've got. Don't go into it timid and passive, get after it!

One rule: don't hold back. No one is going to read what you write in here anyway, just you. If we find something amazing but rough around the edges, we can always fix it up a bit in the final product. If it stinks, we'll throw it out. But for now—write as openly and freely as you can...!!

GETTING STARTED

You know who you are, but your readers don't. Some of these questions are just to get the ideas flowing; we can't include everything, but you should think about each question carefully. Your personal statement is really the first step in the interview—some of the things you write about will come up again in the interview, so you're setting the stage for that conversation.

Even if we don't include all of your answers in your statement, you'll have thought through them which will help prepare you for your interview. Often you can elaborate on features of your statement during your interview. Think of the two (personal statement + interview) as linked; they're a package deal.

Let's start easy; for these answers, just a few words or a few sentences as your answer is fine:

1. Where did you learn of the PA profession?

2. Why not a Doctor, Dentist, Physical Therapist, NP, CRNA, RN, etc.? What research did you do to come to this conclusion?

3. Who supports you the most on your way to being a PA?

4. Who have you shadowed, what did you see, and what advice did they give?

Ok, review #1: Have a specific source: who was it? Your family practice provider? A friend whom you respect? You will be asked, so be prepared to give a specific answer.

Describe how it happened: maybe you liked healthcare but weren't sure which field was right, so you spent a year as a phlebotomist or EKG tech to see different hospital departments? Maybe the PA at your PCP office was the only person to treat you as an adult during adolescence, and that meant a lot to you? Write some details—"show, don't tell".

Now review #2: Specifically, what draws you to the PA profession? What features or responsibilities come together in the PA profession that the others don't have?

Be honest with yourself: "I don't know", "it seems cool", or "I want to be like a doctor" are all unacceptable. Really think about it; why, over all other professions, are you drawn to the PA profession? Ratio of time in school to salary after graduation has no place here. (Note: don't base any decision solely on money!!) How much research did you do about the profession versus others?

It's also good to note, admissions committees don't look favorably on those who are simply applying to PA school because they didn't get into medical/dental school. Even if that's the position you're in, don't include it. They don't want their program to be your "backup plan", and honestly—there's more to you anyway than a missed attempt at medical school…elaborate on the rest of you.

Question #3 looks at your support system. Who do you have in your corner? Who is cheering you on when things get hard? Do you have family/friend support? This is important to assess for incoming students because the courses are hard, and students need a support system to rely on. It also makes you human, not just a name on paper.

Question #4: List any PA you may have shadowed; this provides possible info for your statement, but you can look back to refresh your memory prior to your PA school interview and reference your experiences.

MOTIVATION

Ok, now some harder questions. These might require a few sentences or paragraph. I've offered some suggestions, but don't limit yourself to these. Write your own using the examples just to get you started:

5.   What/who is most important to you? (church, hobbies, pets, spouse/kids/significant other, friends, etc.)

6.   What makes you tick? What gets you up each day? (Solving problems, helping people in need, professional growth, leadership…to name a few?)

7. What are your strongest traits? (leadership, adaptability, talking with people, teaching, understanding difficult concepts, close attention to detail)

8. What are your biggest fears related to school or anything else? Don't forget—no one is reading this but you! (Fear of failing, not amounting to anything, letting your parents/spouse down, keeping up with workload, looking dumb, not getting in to school, repeating past mistakes)

9. What is the weakest part of your application? Is it a lack of prior healthcare experience, suboptimal grades (Organic Chemistry anyone??), overall GPA...identify what might stand out to the committee as a potential drawback to your application?:

Numbers 5, 6 & 8 show you why you do what you do, why you're pursuing PA school. Both positives and negatives, these show you your motivation. We want to support the things/people most important to us while satisfying the things that make us tick and avoiding our biggest fears.

Your answers to number 7 are going to be the hardest to include without sounding like a salesperson. You're not selling, you're showing the real you—when you do, you'll be irresistible. Even though it seems contrived, still mark them down…

Numbers 8 & 9 is difficult to acknowledge, so good for you for writing it out. Just as you need to be prepared to show off your strengths, you also need to defend any weaknesses in your application. While it most likely won't be included in your statement, it might come up in interviews, so we need to address it privately right now so you're at least aware of it and can anticipate potential questions from the application committee and prepare for possible discussion.

FORMATIVE EXPERIENCES

We're all influenced by the unique experiences we've had. That's what makes us unique. They are ever-changing too. My answers to these questions would be different now than when I applied to PA school—as time has passed, I've had additional experiences since then. We're constantly molded by events that happen to us over time.

This is where we get away from the superficial and really see who you are. This is where you can look at major life events, births/deaths, family events, military service, real world situations, and many others as the stuff that makes you YOU. (I know, total cheese...but it's true for this purpose.)

Many writing resources talk about storytelling in writing application essays. This is very true, because it hits our focus: it helps you stand out as an individual, but also draws the reader in. Wouldn't you rather read a story with a beginning, middle, end than a list of facts?

When I was 17, I went on a backpacking trip. I had the blessing to spend 30 days in the mountains of Colorado learning about leadership and team building, which by itself could make for a good story. While the experience was amazing, it was augmented by something that happened right before I left for the trip: a 10 minute encounter with a homeless man one random night.

I don't know what was so striking about the encounter—nothing was particularly moving about the words that were exchanged, but rather the whole experience together was quite life-changing.

I was buying some things for my upcoming backpacking trip from a camping store and had thrown the stuff in the back seat of my gently used car. A big 40-50-year-old guy in an old blue satin jacket walked toward me. The kind of jacket that should have a baseball team logo on the back with striped trim and snaps down the front. He had thick smudged glasses with frames that could have been two decades old.

"Hey man…?"

I looked up. Embarrassingly, the first thing I thought about was the safety of the $200 worth of camping gear I had just put in the back seat.

"Um, me?"

He walked toward me, extended his thick, calloused, dirty hand. I shook it.

"Do you, uh….can you spare some cash?"

Selfishly, I didn't want to spend any more money. I had just bought a bunch of stuff, paid cash, and shoved the change in my pockets. I didn't know how much I had.

"Just a little bit if you've got it…whatever you can spare." he said, kind of trailing off.

I reached into my pocket and pulled out what I had left: a $20 and a few $1 bills. I got nervous—if I gave him the few $1, that would be super cheap since I obviously had more, but the $20 was (at that point, still being selfish) to buy Burger King on the way home for myself.

We both looked down at what was in my hand, then looked at each other. The pain in his eyes was apparent: he looked weary, embarrassed to even be asking, and hungry.

"What's your name, sir?" I asked.

"Jim. The name's Jim."

With just his name, I was struck by how stupid it was to be perseverating over $20 when I had just spent 10x that amount.

"Well, here you go Jim, get something to eat" I said as I handed him everything in my hand.

He looked down at roughly $23, took it, then grabbed me in a huge hug.

He didn't let go for what seemed like an eternity, and when he did he had tears rolling down his face.

"I've got two little kids that are hungry and with this I can feed them tonight AND tomorrow."

I immediately felt so ashamed of the fact that I almost didn't give it to him in order to get dinner on the way home (my usual two 9-piece Chicken Tenders with barbeque sauce). Although Burger King *can* be delicious, it couldn't come close to seeing this guy ecstatic about providing something for his family. Plus, I had a full pantry at home, but this guy might have nothing...

I asked if he needed a ride somewhere nearby. He asked to be taken for a few blocks if that was okay with me (I am not recommending this...!!).

I wondered if I'd drop him off at an apartment, a house, or a homeless shelter. The whole way he told me about losing his job and not being able to find work. After a few blocks and a few turns, he told me to stop up ahead. We literally stopped under an overpass where he shook my hand again.

"Thanks man...God bless you!" he said, then came in for another hug, this time more awkward as I was tethered by my seatbelt and he was a grown man half in-half out of the passenger seat.

He got out and shut the door. I could hear him yell "Daddy's home…and we're gonna EAT!" I looked over my shoulder out the back window as I drove away to see two small kids walk up to him grab onto his legs…just as excited as he was.

I drove home in silence—no radio, nothing. Just thinking of the man who literally lived under an overpass with his family, who was thrilled to be serve his family food for 2 days with $23 while I drove home in my own car to a house in the suburbs.

I knew in my head that homelessness was real, but by witnessing it firsthand that night, I felt it. I was never going to solve the reality of homelessness, but I helped that night. And I knew I made the right choice to use my cash to help rather than hoard it for myself. I learned a major driving factor of my life yet to come: I really want to help people at every opportunity.

As I was on that trip, I couldn't shake the memory of that night. I returned with a renewed sense of purpose, so I naturally wanted to include the experience in my personal statement somehow, since it was a significant experience for me. But was "helping people" enough?

My experience with Jim left a lasting impression on me, but I obviously couldn't write the whole story in my personal statement—I'd reduce it down to something that sends the theme of the experience, but I could do it one of two ways: I could play it safe or send a strong message about what I learned from that encounter.

Like mentioned earlier, there are things that draw all of us to the PA profession—helping people, making a difference, etc. Focusing on these directly isn't really different, but a story or message that touches on it in a compelling way can get the point across in an engaging way.

So which way reads better?:

Safe: "I learned as a teenager how rewarding helping others less fortunate than me can be."

Stronger: "A chance encounter with a homeless man taught me I desperately need to help others; I see people all around me in need from illness, poverty, and circumstances. I can't solve all of these, but being a PA will allow me to positively impact one of them."

Strongest: "My 10 minute conversation with a homeless man was a punch in the gut; it rattled my privileged upbrining to make me bound and determined to make a difference with my life."

The safe sentence is fluffy and nice (and true), the stronger sentence is a little better and descriptive, but the strong sentences send a better message. It shows motivation, determiniation, desire, and a calling to the profession. It also leads to a story; a few lines to draw the reader in. You can tell the rest in your interview. Go the strong route; it's a fight, remember?

YOUR TURN

Similar to my exchange with Jim, write out details of your stories.

What are the 3 most formative/defining experiences of your life. Elaborate. Why were they special? Why did they define your life from that point forward? This could be anything from a birth or death of a family member, scary/traumatic experience, etc. You're not going to include all of these in your final copy, but once you start thinking about them, it might spur on additional memories, so you'll pick from the best one.

1.

2.

3.

Look at all 3 together; what themes do you see between these events? Are there any similarities between them? If so, note them. If not, no problem. What is the theme for each individual event?

1.

2.

3.

For each: write a "strong" sentence to sum up your experiences.

First

Second

Third

COMPETITION

So...you know you have competition with other applicants. You know who they are: you've been sitting next to them in prerequisite classes this whole time. Same classes, same majors. Some have even gotten better grades than you. But they're still *not* you. So what makes you different?

Why do you deserve a seat in this class? (Be honest....you're the bomb, so write down why!!)

Thinking about it differently, how have your formative experiences set you up for success as a PA student and eventually a practicing PA? Make the connection for your reader: how do those themes translate into you being a good provider?

Finally, what do you want the admissions committee to know about you that isn't covered elsewhere? The rest of your application is pretty dry with grades, achievements, and demographics, so what else can you add that hasn't been covered?

10 KEY POINTS TO REMEMBER

Congratulations!! The hard part is done! You've gotten some good stuff out and written down, now we just need to assemble your thoughts in a compelling way.

First, here are **10 things you need to remember as you assemble your essay**:

1. <u>Consider your audience.</u> Don't confuse this with writing what they want to hear, but rather remember who is reading your statement. They're a committee member, usually voluntary, who has to sift through hundreds of applications. If you waste time over-developing your tone or situation, you'll lose their attention as they look through the stack of other essays to read. But you have to keep in mind who will be assessing your work.

2. <u>Write conversationally, but professionally.</u> If you write your statement as you would talk in your interview, it will likely flow better. You can go back through and remove contractions to make sure it sounds professional. You might even use the recipe below to dictate the essay into your phone or word processor, then go back and edit. Try it, you might be surprised at the outcome! Writing formally is a great skill—but don't forget, this is a conversation about you, not a journal article.

3. <u>Don't waste time with needless details.</u> Space is limited; the max character count is 5000, which is actually a blessing because it forces you to get to the point. This helps the reader as well: come out swinging and get to it. (Remember, this includes punctuation, spaces, and paragraph breaks!)

4. <u>Show aspects of yourself that aren't developed in other areas of your application.</u> This is not the place to list all your achievements, there's another spot for that in your application. Don't waste your characters on things that are already listed

elsewhere. Everyone has unique characteristics that don't "fit" in the rest of the application; show them off here!

5. <u>Don't dwell on weaknesses</u>; you can touch on them if they end up being pertinent to your story, but don't dwell. You'll have that opportunity to discuss at your interview. As noted earlier, it is valuable for you to know and recognize your weaknesses. It will allow you to acknowledge them and mentally prepare to respond to any issues that are brought up in your interview. If your grades were rough one semester because of a life event, use it. If you changed your major part way through and the workload was harder than you thought, show how you adapted and overcame. Just don't feel the need to spend your whole statement making up for your weaknesses.

6. <u>Don't try too hard to be funny</u>; comedy reads differently to different audiences, and almost always it needs to be within some other context (usually personality). I constantly get in awkward situations trying to be funny in group text messages, but my wife just says "no, no...that makes no sense...don't send that". Bless her heart. (I pretend it's because the humor doesn't read well, but she doesn't think I'm that funny!)

7. <u>Avoid religion and politics</u>. The only exception to this rule is if you're applying to a faith-based institution...then religion is ok. Politics however...save that for debates with your classmates!

8. <u>Don't assume the reader can place things as relevant.</u> Sometimes we draw conclusions in our mind that seem logical to us, but someone reading might not have the extra information you have needed to tie ideas together. If you leave it up to the reader to draw conclusions or connections, you run the risk of confusing them, so draw conclusions for them.

9. <u>Don't pretend to be someone else.</u> This is a representation of you, so don't play a character you think they want to

see. They'll meet you in your interview, so they'll find out sooner or later if you're putting up a front. Having said this, you want to put your best foot forward. Think of a first date: you don't put everything on the table right away, but (hopefully) you're being authentic with the side of you that you're sharing. Same for your essay, application, and interview. Put your best foot forward, but remain true to who you are.

10. <u>SPELLING AND GRAMMAR ERRORS ARE UNACCEPTABLE!!!</u> Please, please, please proofread your statement, then have someone else proofread it as well. Ideally, this person will know you well and can tell if it adequately represents you. It's awkward though, for sure…you're opening yourself up for criticism, so if it's just too much, find someone else you know less or look online. There are several PAs who offer to review your personal statement (usually for a fee), but they can have some valuable feedback as well without knowing you personally.

If all else fails, send it my way and I'll read it. If I have suggestions, I'm happy to share them, but beware—I'm not afraid to share opinions. It's in your best interest though…! Shoot me an email at chris@pastartup.co, or send me a tweet too if you want: @PAStartupDOTco

Refer back to these 10 things as you put the pieces together. You'll want to make sure you're following these along the way.

ASSEMBLY OF YOUR STATEMENT

When I was in 7th grade, I made brownies with a small group as part of a class project. None of us had ever cooked or baked on our own before, so we added all the ingredients together and microwaved it all at once. It did NOT turn out well. Inedible nastiness.

Your essay is like a pan of brownies. We need to follow some steps to make sure these brownies turn out perfect. We have to be strategic where we put each element. The chances of the admissions committee reading each and every word is low, so we need the theme of your essay to show up in key spots on the page.

Here's an overview of the "recipe", although like cooking, you have some latitude. But in my opinion, staying close to this guide will yield the best flow of your content while placing key features strategically within the document. This will seem different than collegiate-level writing, and it is. It's not a research paper, it's your story. Use this as a guide; it doesn't matter how many paragraphs you end up with so long as you stay within the 5000 character count.

STARTING "RECIPE"

1. Best formative experience strong sentence. Key features (themes) of your experiences

2. Why you deserve seat

3. Strengths/motivation

4. Other info not included in rest of essay. Also, why PA rather than other types of jobs (need to see not second choice)

5. Summary

BREAKING IT DOWN

There have been a lot of studies done on resumes and statistics gathered on how hiring managers sift through resumes. Since your personal narrative is basically your resume, we want to format it in a similar way.

Statistically, people read the beginning of the first paragraph and a few lines of the last paragraph and skim the middle. If that's true about your essay (and I can attest it's about right), that leaves you 6 seconds to make a good impression. That's not much, but plenty for us to draw the reader in for more. Keep in mind, these don't necessarily have to be grouped 5 paragraphs--use your judgement, but this will help you establish a flow through the page.

First Section
Since we have 6 seconds (ok, that might not be scientifically proven, but it illustrates my point!), we need to start off with a bang. Since the name of the game is to stand out and capitalize on your unique-ness, need to start with your starred "strongest" formative sentence. Which was your strongest sentence? Look on page 26—if it's not written in an appropriate format, rewrite it here if needed:

These experiences naturally set you up to start to tell a story. Again, you have to keep it fairly brief, so provide an overview of the situation and add the themes you identified between these and add any supporting info to help the story.

If these feel too "buzzwordy", you can even comment on this directly: "All applicants want to help, but my experience is unique because…" or something similar.

It's common to try to hit medical buzzwords throughout your essay to show you belong in the PA profession, but I disagree. By making your statement conversational (while professional), downplaying buzzwords will make you stand out more. It seems counterintuitive, but if a personal statement is devoid of buzzwords, it can cause the reader pause longer to see what's actually written. That's the moment you can draw the reader in.

Also, if something you write might raise a question, answer it for the reader. "My encounter with a homeless man was life changing" would be followed by the reader saying "why?", so you need to answer the question for them: "I saw there are people in need everywhere, but since I cannot solve all problems, I can focus on one: healthcare."

Second Section

Follow this with a section on why you deserve a seat in the class. This is from page 27 where we tied the themes of your formative experiences to why you'll be a good PA provider. Remember to draw conclusions for the reader, don't expect them to link your experience and why it will make you a good PA. It's fine to be direct—you can even say "when I think about my key formative experiences, the theme that stands out the most is…"

Take the reader further into the themes you drew between your key formative experiences. What traits do you have that other applicants don't have? The first time through go ahead and write with contractions and use normal conversational tone.

Third Section
Move on to strengths and motivation from pages 15 and 16. Elaborate on why these strengths naturally set you up to be a great PA, and even so far as to why you should beat out others for your seat. Maybe your class load demonstrates you can handle a heavy schedule? Maybe you graduated at the top of your class?

Fourth Section
Include things that aren't elsewhere in your application. It gets this information in front of the applications committee in a way the rest of your application might not allow. Perhaps you published a paper or did some great community service: illustrate your experience here.

Also, touch on why you chose the PA profession over other allied health fields. This should be present somewhere in your statement so the committee knows you're focused on being a PA specifically. If your formative experience included this, don't worry about trying to include it again...it just needs to be in there somewhere.

Final Section
Review the high points. The first sentence of your last section should be the second most moving sentence of your essay (the first line of the first paragraph was the biggest "bang"): after the first line of the first paragraph, this is likely the second place the reader will skim. Usually, you can reiterate your main point, then summarize what you've said throughout your various paragraphs, followed by a closing line. You can even directly address your competition—"I know there are numerous strong applicants, but I will make a good PA because..." I know it seems silly, after years of writing on a college level to finish your statement with a "conclusion paragraph" like we did in 6th grade--but remember, if the reader is pressed for time, they'll read the beginning and the end, so it gives you the chance to get those key points in front of them.

This last part isn't a literary concept or anything, but it makes a difference: end your essay with an open-ended sentence or question. Something that naturally leaves the reader with no choice but to offer you an interview:

"After my experience with X, how can I do anything else?"
"I can't wait to be a PA"
"I look forward to a career as a PA-C"

EDITING

There you have it; put this all down in a Word document (or any other writing app). Look for misspellings, change contractions to their appropriate format for graduate-level writing (is that "uncontracted"??), and look for any grammar issues or punctuation errors.

This next step is important: save it and close it. Don't look at it anymore. Take a walk, enjoy life. Leave it alone for a day or two. Exercise, go out for appetizers— completely forget about your essay.

After a little vacation from the world of essay writing, come back and read it with fresh eyes. Did it grab your attention? How does it flow? Any glaring errors that jump out? Fix them—print it and make marks on paper so you can read all the way through without stopping to make changes, then make them all at once in the computer. Then walk away again. Repeat the above.

The third time through, re-read with the same goals, but by now hopefully you're not finding much. Anything not sitting quite right? Maybe your choice of words is weird somewhere, or one section is clunky. Try some alternative solutions one more time. Maybe you find your original way flows the best; trying other ways can convince you to keep the original.

Finally, send it on to someone for review. Parent, sibling, best friend, spouse, significant other...anyone who knows you is the best option since you're trying to provide an accurate representation of YOU. They don't necessarily need to be an English major, although another set of eyes looking for sentence structure, grammar, and spelling errors isn't a bad thing either.

I strongly encourage you to put yourself out there to someone you know, even if it's intimidating or awkward. I know it stinks,

Writing Your PA School Application Essay

but it will be most beneficial to you. If you really don't have that trusted someone, search online for a few PA blogs that offer essay proofreading….and again, if you don't have anyone or can't pay, send it my way and I'll look at it for free: chris@pastartup.co. Subject: Workbook review.

PLEASE keep in mind; any feedback you're given by your reader isn't an attack on you as a person, but rather how accurately your writing reflects you and the message it sends. We all want you to succeed, so don't take it personally…! Review and address their concerns if needed, then relax. You're done! Mark it off your applications checklist!

Strong work. You made it through! Now submit that application and let me know how things go. I can't wait to hear where you're interviewing, how the process has gone, and most importantly—I can't wait to call you a colleague!!

Take care,
Chris

P.S. I have other guides in the works, but they take time to produce. If you'd like to hear about new guides when they're released, head over to PAStartup.co and opt in to my email list. I won't bug you excessively…I promise! I'll just keep you up to date when new guides or podcasts are released.

Also, if you'd be so kind as to not share this book with others, but please direct them to Amazon or PAStartup.co to purchase their own. Thanks much!

BONUS INTERVIEW QUESTIONS

Here are some common interview questions; this is by no means exhaustive, but you'll see the style of questioning and can start to plan on how to answer them.

Interview questions aren't yes/no type questions by design; you need to anticipate some of the common things they'll ask. There are obvious ones like: What is a PA? How do PAs differ from Physicians? Do a little reading before your interview to get up to speed with current issues with PAs; the American Academy of Physician Assistants (AAPA.org) is a great place to start.

The 12 questions below are some of the more difficult ones to answer as they are very subjective:

1. Give an example of a time you sacrificed for others?
2. How do you handle problem solving?
3. How would you handle a difficult patient?
4. Who are the significant role models in your life?
5. Where do you see yourself practicing—rural, underserved, specialty care, etc.?
6. Where do you see yourself in 10 years?
7. What is the single most defining moment of your life thus far?
8. What is your worst trait? (Don't be too hard on yourself, we're only human. I'm chronically late. Just figure out a way to joke about it—"At least I'm ready for medical time!")
9. What would you do if you were put on the waitlist?
10. What are your plans if you don't get in this year?
11. How many schools are you applying to?
12. Why don't you want to be a Physician?

ABOUT THE AUTHOR

Chris Darst, MPAS, PA-C is a husband and father of 3 beautiful girls ages 12, 10, and 8. When he can't be with them, he is the head PA for a Cardiothoracic Surgery practice in the Midwest, usually dreaming of mountains and oceans, neither of which are close by.

Chris@pastartup.co
Twitter: @PAStartupDOTco
Facebook: @PAStartup.co

DISCLAIMER

The information contained in this guide is for informational purposes only.

This workbook provides an outline for assembling your PA School Application Essay as directed by CASPA, but does not in any way guarantee success related to your PA School application, chances of an interview, or acceptance to an accredited Physician Assistant Program.

I am also not a lawyer or accountant, and therefore any legal or financial advice given or inferred in this guide (or other materials published by Enlighten Medical Media, LLC) is solely my opinion based on experience.

No part of this publication shall be reproduced, transmitted, or sold in whole or in part in any form, without the prior written consent of the author. Any/all trademarks and registered trademarks appearing in this guide are the property of their respective owners.

Purchasing, downloading, and/or reading this guide acknowledges the author and Enlighten Medical Media, LLC and PAStartup.co are not responsible for the success or failure of your PA School application but rather or this and other resources as a template and outline guide for your essay production.

© 2017 Enlighten Medical Media, LLC

NOTES:

NOTES:

NOTES:

NOTES:

NOTES:

NOTES:

www.ingramcontent.com/pod-product-compliance
Lightning Source LLC
LaVergne TN
LVHW041309080426
835510LV00009B/927